BLOOD PRESSURE

**Questions
you
have
...Answers
you
need**

Other Books in This Series
From the People's Medical Society

Alzheimer's & Dementia: Questions You Have . . . Answers You Need

Arthritis: Questions You Have . . . Answers You Need

Asthma: Questions You Have . . . Answers You Need

Back Pain: Questions You Have . . . Answers You Need

Cholesterol & Triglycerides: Questions You Have . . . Answers You Need

Depression: Questions You Have . . . Answers You Need

Diabetes: Questions You Have . . . Answers You Need

Hearing Loss: Questions You Have . . . Answers You Need

Prostate: Questions You Have . . . Answers You Need

Stroke: Questions You Have . . . Answers You Need

Vitamins and Minerals: Questions You Have . . . Answers You Need

Your Eyes: Questions You Have . . . Answers You Need

Your Heart: Questions You Have . . . Answers You Need

BLOOD PRESSURE

Questions you have ...Answers you need

By
The Staff of the
People's Medical Society

≡People's Medical Society®

Allentown, Pennsylvania

The People's Medical Society is a nonprofit consumer health organization dedicated to the principles of better, more responsive and less expensive medical care. Organized in 1983, the People's Medical Society puts previously unavailable medical information into the hands of consumers so that they can make informed decisions about their own health care.

Membership in the People's Medical Society is $20 a year and includes a subscription to the *People's Medical Society Newsletter.* For information, write to the People's Medical Society, 462 Walnut Street, Allentown, PA 18102, or call 610-770-1670.

This and other People's Medical Society publications are available for quantity purchase at discount. Contact the People's Medical Society for details.

Many of the designations used by manufacturers and sellers to distinguish their products are claimed as trademarks. Where those designations appear in this book and the People's Medical Society was aware of a trademark claim, the designations have been printed in initial capital letters (e.g., Procardia).

© 1996 by the People's Medical Society
Printed in the United States of America

Library of Congress Cataloging-in-Publication Data
Blood pressure : questions you have, answers you need / by the
    staff of the People's Medical Society.
        p.   cm.
    Includes index.
    ISBN 1-882606-61-2
    1. Hypertension—Popular works.   2. Blood-pressure—
Popular works.   I. People's Medical Society (U.S.)
RC685.H8B3955   1996
616.1'32—dc20   95-46873
                                                         CIP

        6 7 8 9 0
First printing, February 1996

INTRODUCTION

Fifty million Americans have high blood pressure, or hypertension. More than 35,000 deaths each year are directly attributed to it. It is *the* most common chronic medical condition, yet only half of those who have it know it. It's called America's *silent killer* because most people who have it have no visible symptoms.

When the People's Medical Society published the first edition of this book in 1984, our impetus was the mail we received from members and consumers who wanted the unbiased facts about the causes, treatments and controversies surrounding hypertension. We reviewed the existing books and pamphlets available to consumers about blood pressure and found that most had a bias. Sometimes the bias was the author's—a physician who treats the condition only one way, ignoring other acceptable treatments. Other publications were skewed to specific products—suggesting the use of a particular drug from a particular manufacturer, for instance.

What was missing was an easy-to-read, understandable book that not only explained all the possible causes of high (and low) blood pressure but also the whole range of treatments available. That's why we decided to write this book.

This latest edition of *Blood Pressure: Questions You Have...Answers You Need* is completely updated, providing you with the latest research on hypertension, the good news and the bad. We cover conventional as well as alternative treatments for blood pressure problems. And we cover them in ways that will allow you to have an informed and useful interaction with your health-care provider.

Like all People's Medical Society books, *Blood Pressure: Questions You Have...Answers You Need* is an information tool designed to help you take charge of your health and health care. Our goal at the People's Medical Society is not to tell you what to do, but instead to give you the information to make the decision yourself. And you can do that with the full range of information you'll find in the pages that follow.

Charles B. Inlander
President
People's Medical Society

BLOOD PRESSURE

**Questions
you
have
...Answers
you
need**

Terms printed in boldface can be found in the glossary, beginning on page 84. Only the first mention of the word in the text will be boldfaced.

We have tried to use male and female pronouns in an egalitarian manner throughout the book. Any imbalance in usage has been in the interest of readability.

Q: What exactly *is* **blood pressure**?

A: It's the force of your blood's trip from your heart to and through the rest of your arterial and **vascular system**. When your heart beats—when that portion of your heart called the **left ventricle** contracts—oxygenated blood is literally shot into your arteries.

In its travels through your body, your blood presses against the walls of the blood vessels it's passing through. The vessels stretch and contract to maintain blood flow. If the vessels are narrowed, increasing the resistance to blood flow, blood pressure rises.

When it comes to measuring blood pressure and expressing it in numbers everybody can understand, there are two sets of readings. When the left ventricle contracts, and the blood's force against the vessel walls is at its greatest strength, you have what is called **systolic** pressure. After that contraction, when the heart is more or less in its resting phase, the blood pressure is lower.

This resting or relaxation pressure—the pressure in the arteries just before the next heartbeat—is known as the **diastolic** pressure.

Blood pressure readings, then, come in two numbers. For example, 120/80 (expressed as "120 over 80") or 150/95, and so on. The first number is the systolic, while the second number is the diastolic. The difference between the two readings is known as the **pulse pressure**.

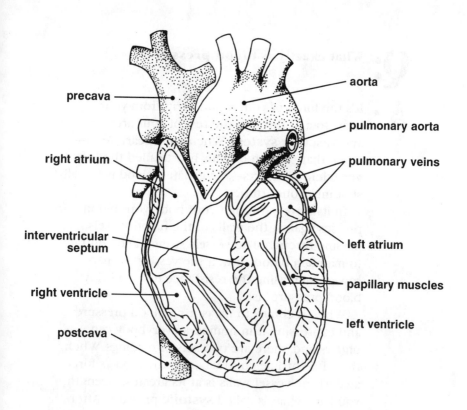

precava

aorta

pulmonary aorta

right atrium

pulmonary veins

interventricular septum

left atrium

right ventricle

papillary muscles

postcava

left ventricle

Q: Which of the blood pressure numbers is more important—the systolic or the diastolic?

A: Both are of interest and concern to doctors. Traditionally, the emphasis was on the diastolic, but current guidelines recognize systolic blood pressure as a defining factor of equal importance in the medical evaluation of blood pressure.

Q: What is **normal blood pressure?**

A: "Normal" is always a relative term when it comes to the way human beings function. Taking body function measurements isn't like taking a history exam: There aren't any "correct" answers or "perfect" scores. A lot depends on a whole host of conditions.

By most accounts, a reading of about 120-129 systolic over 80-84 diastolic is "normal." But you'd be hard pressed to find anybody with exactly 120/80 pressure, or with exactly 120/80 all the time. The 120/80 measurement is an average of a pretty wide range of readings. Various times of the day, activities or emotional states can raise or lower the reading without being a sign of anything wrong.

Q: How do you get those numbers—120 over 80, and such—anyway? And what's "mm" and "Hg"? I've seen those abbreviations used with blood pressure readings, but I don't know what they stand for.

A: Those numbers are derived from readings taken with the standard blood-pressure-measuring device, called a **sphygmomanometer** (pronounced *sfig-mo-muh-NOM-i-tur*—it's a toughie, all right). If you've ever had a physical examination, you've met up with a sphygmomanometer. Most people refer to it simply as a **blood pressure cuff**.

The way it works is this: A wide band, or cuff, is wrapped around your upper arm. The cuff is then inflated by air pressure. At the same time, the air pressure pushes a column of liquid mercury (*Hg* is the scientist's abbreviation for mercury) up along a numbered scale that is measured in millimeters (usually abbreviated as *mm*).

A stethoscope is placed against your arm's artery, known as the **brachial artery**. When the cuff has been inflated enough to cut off circulation to the lower part of the brachial artery, the person listening through the stethoscope (which is placed against the artery at the crook of the arm) will hear no sound. As the pressure is slowly released, the cuff loosens, the blood begins to flow again into the lower artery, and the column of mercury falls. At the point when the stethoscope can pick up the tapping of the heartbeat in the artery, the millimeter level of mercury indicates a figure approximately equal to the systolic pressure. Soon, as the pressure in the cuff is further released, the beating sound disappears. The number on the millimeter scale at that point is approximately that of the diastolic pressure.

So if your blood pressure is 120/80, or 120 mm Hg/80 mm Hg, what that means is that your systolic pressure was detected, pinpointed and measured when the column of mercury was at a height of 120 millimeters, and your diastolic pressure was detected, pinpointed and measured when the column of mercury was at a height of 80 millimeters. The numbers merely represent a convenient method of noting and comparing blood pressures.

Q: Are blood pressure readings with a sphygmomanometer accurate?

A: They're close but not perfect. While other, more accurate measurement methods exist, they are far too complicated and invasive for general office or home use. For the most part, a sphygmomanometer reading is actually somewhat lower than the true arterial pressure.

Another problem with this indirect method of determining blood pressure is that you can get incorrect readings if you don't do the procedure just right. For example, if you don't pump the cuff tight enough—and, thus, don't entirely collapse the brachial artery—you'll get a reading that's too low. The same goes if you let the air out too quickly, or if you use an adult-size cuff on children or grown-ups with very thin arms.

You might get a false high reading if a person's arm is too thick for the standard cuff. That's why some obese people who don't have **high blood pressure**, or **hypertension**, seem to—it's not their blood pressure, it's the inadequate size of the cuff that's providing the false reading. And your home reading could be way off if you take your pressure with your arm resting on a table or in some other such elevated position—the cuff ought to be at heart level, and the best way to do that is if the arm is kept down at your side.

In today's booming self-care market, most new, low-cost blood-pressure-measuring devices are not the mercury column type of sphygmomanometer. Instead they have gauges or digital readouts. While the mercury column types are still considered the best, most accurate and most durable, they are a bit more complicated to use without help. The new kids on the blood pressure block can do well enough if they are, first, well-made and, second, taken care of. And, perhaps, occasionally serviced, if possible.

And don't forget to ask your health practitioner if his or her sphygmomanometer has been checked for accuracy and serviced lately. Incidents of office sphygmomanometers being way off—and thus affecting treatment options—are more common than you might think.

Q: **I'm usually nervous when I visit my doctor. Can my anxiety affect my blood pressure reading?**

A: Yes. A doctor-induced case of the jitters can cause your blood pressure to climb. This tendency for blood pressure to rise in the doctor's office— although it's usually normal the rest of the time— is called **white-coat hypertension**. This type of hypertension can occur at any age and in both sexes, but it seems to be slightly more common in people over age 60, according to the *American Journal of Hypertension*.

Labile hypertension is the name given to high blood pressure that fluctuates—for whatever the reason—and is not persistent. **Sustained hypertension** means you have it all the time. If not taken care of, labile hypertension can become persistent and health endangering.

Q: Back to white-coat hypertension—what can a person do about it? Health-care practitioners have to measure blood pressure, right?

A: Usually if you have a high initial reading your doctor will measure your blood pressure several times over a few days—or even a couple of times in one visit, for the simple reason that a single reading does not take into account blood pressure's normal, everyday ups and downs or the effects of stress. Further, measuring blood pressure at home to supplement readings taken in the doctor's office can help eliminate the distortion produced by the white-coat effect and help determine if you have true hypertension. In the somewhat tongue-in-cheek words of a *Lancet* article, "The measurement of blood pressure is much too serious to be left to physicians."

Q: Can you tell me more about home blood pressure monitoring?

A: Certainly. Self-monitoring holds two essential potential advantages. Not only does it help determine whether a person has white-coat hypertension, but it also allows for multiple readings taken over long periods of time. True, there is ample opportunity for errors in home readings—perhaps more so than with physician readings—but these errors can be all but avoided by the use of automatic devices.

In short, exclusive reliance on either method—in-office readings or self-monitoring—is not recommended.

Q: **Okay. Now can you tell me more about manual blood pressure devices versus automatic models?**

A: In general, the manual cuff requires a bit more work because you need to learn how to inflate the cuff, listen for the heartbeat and read the blood pressure gauge. The automatic models do all the work for you.

But before we go into the pluses and minuses of each, let's take a look at the different types of blood-pressure-monitoring devices. Here's what Cathey Pinckney and Edward R. Pinckney, M.D., writing in *Do-It-Yourself Medical Testing,* have to say about the options. There are:

- Devices that use mercury that rises and falls within a glass tube and require a stethoscope to listen for the pulse sounds

- Aneroid devices that convert mm Hg into figures on a gauge or circular dial face (similar to a thermometer). Some of these require a stethoscope, and some do not—the latter instead use a built-in microphone in place of the stethoscope.

- Digital devices that directly display the diastolic and systolic pressures

- Automatic devices that inflate the cuff to the proper level and then release the air at the proper time. Some even produce a printed read-out of the person's blood pressure and pulse.

- Devices that measure blood pressure via cuffs wrapped around a finger or a wrist and that often inflate automatically

Q: So what are the pros and cons of each?

A: The mercury type is the most accurate but is also the most difficult to use. The automatic varieties are easier to use—but they are more expensive and have poorer accuracy rates.

Q: If I decide to go with an automatic sphyg-momanometer, do I have a choice of types?

A: Yes. The automatic models include digital devices that display the systolic and diastolic pressures—and sometimes the pulse rate—directly. As we just mentioned, there are also some new sphygmoma-nometers that automatically inflate the cuff to the proper level and then release the air at the proper time, either displaying the results digitally or printing a record. These printed results are a great way to provide a record for your practitioner. Many of the latest models don't even require you to roll up your sleeve—again, as we mentioned, they measure your blood pressure from a cuff around your wrist.

The authors of *Do-It-Yourself Medical Testing* suggest that, before buying any blood pressure device, you try it out in the pharmacy to make sure you can use it easily and properly. You should also try out two or three of the same model as well as a few different brands to see whether the readings are nearly identical. After you purchase a device, it is also a good idea to take your sphygmomanometer to your practitioner's office and compare the readings of the two devices.

Q: You've told me about a lot of different kinds of sphygmomanometers, but what can you say about the at-home blood pressure monitor that fits over a finger?

A: You may want to skip this device until manufacturers work out the kinks. Opt instead for the style with the wrist or arm cuff. The reason for this cautionary note is that a small study found that these finger monitors produced blood pressure measurements that fell within 4 mm Hg of traditional sphygmomanometer readings in *less than* 25 percent of cases.

Q: Aside from these home blood pressure monitors, are there any other ways to supplement my practitioner's blood pressure measurements?

A: Clinical measurements of blood pressure can be supplemented not only by home measurements but also by **ambulatory monitoring**.

Q: What is ambulatory monitoring?

A: Ambulatory monitoring is a technique in which multiple blood pressure readings are taken by a personal monitor over a period of time while the person conducts everyday, normal activities. First developed more than 30 years ago, ambulatory monitoring has made significant technological strides of late.

Becoming increasingly available are monitors that take up to 100 blood pressure readings over 24 hours while people go about their normal activities. Although studies have shown that ambulatory monitors can help distinguish between white-coat hypertension and true high blood pressure, the monitors are expensive and impractical for many people.

Q: You've explained using at-home and ambulatory devices to complement my doctor's readings, but what about those machines I see in my drugstore and supermarket? Do they work?

A: They may work after you deposit your quarters— but you cannot always trust their readings. Some studies have found that the blood-pressure-cuff computers found in many stores are incorrect more than 60 percent of the time, compared with readings taken with a sphygmomanometer. Clearly, then, the moral is not to rely on solely one reading in determining whether you have—or don't have—high blood pressure.

Q: Okay, now I know how to have my blood pressure measured. But when is a blood pressure reading considered high blood pressure?

A: As we said earlier, it's a fuzzy area. According to the medical experts, when blood pressure remains at 140/90 over a period of time (usually at least two readings over three days, or after several hours' rest) that's high blood pressure, or hypertension.

In the past, the medical guidelines for diagnosing high blood pressure were more relaxed—that is, set higher—for older folks, and people over 40 were considered in danger if their readings were 160/95 or higher. However, current medical wisdom holds that the cutoff for normal blood pressure levels should be independent of age—in fact, maybe even stricter for older people, since their bodies are more vulnerable to damage from high blood pressure.

The medical profession has also recently replaced its designations of **mild**, **moderate** and **severe hypertension** with a new system of levels, or stages.

Q: Can you tell me more? What are these levels?

A: **Optimal blood pressure** is defined as a systolic blood pressure less than 120 mm Hg and a diastolic blood pressure less than 80 mm Hg. Normal blood pressure is considered to be a systolic reading between 120 and 129 mm Hg and a diastolic reading between 80 and 84 mm Hg. Individuals with a systolic reading between

130 and 139 mm Hg and a diastolic reading between 85 and 89 mm Hg are designated as having **high normal blood pressure**. Individuals with a systolic reading between 140 and 159 mm Hg and a diastolic reading between 90 and 99 mm Hg are designated as having **stage 1 hypertension**; a systolic reading between 160 and 179 mm Hg and a diastolic reading between 100 and 109 mm Hg as **stage 2**; a systolic reading between 180 and 209 mm Hg and a diastolic reading between 110 and 119 mm Hg as **stage 3**; and a systolic reading greater than 210 or a diastolic reading greater than 120 as **stage 4**. (See chart on page 27.)

Q: Is high blood pressure a disease?

A: Definitely.

Q: What causes it?

A: Here's an answer you're going to hear a lot during the course of this book: Nobody knows for sure. It may be due to one thing, or it may have "multifactorial etiology"—scientists' lingo for lots of different causes and reasons. Heredity is one factor, although that only explains transmission, not cause. Diseases of the kidney are prime culprits. The brain chemical acetylcholine has been linked to hypertension, as has something called the natriuretic hormone. **Sleep apnea**—a sudden stoppage of breathing during the night—may cause high blood pressure in older men (although it might be the other way around; nobody knows for sure). Environmental conditions have also been implicated. It could be all or one or none—always, sometimes or never. That's what makes high blood pressure so tough to fight and to make generalities about—and to write inflexible prescriptions for.

Q: Is high blood pressure a common disease?

A: It sure is—somewhere around 50 million Americans, give or take. But only about half of those who have it know they have it.

Q: How can people not know they have high blood pressure? What are the symptoms?

A: That's the point—there are hardly any symptoms at all. And when those few that do exist turn up, it's usually only after the blood pressure is very high already. That's why they call it the silent killer. It's one of nature's little jokes on humans, but about the only way to know if you have high blood pressure is to find it out when you have your pressure checked. Or when you keel over from a **stroke**. That's the drastic way of finding out—it won't help you very much, but it'll answer your next of kin's questions.

For the record, the American Heart Association (AHA) provides these heart-stopping statistics:

- High blood pressure is implicated in many of the deaths and disabilities resulting from strokes. Strokes killed 143,640 people in the United States in 1992, the latest year for which complete statistics are available. Nearly 36,000 more lives were lost because of high blood pressure or hypertensive disease.

- Nearly 58 million Americans have one or more forms of heart or blood vessel disease.

- In 1992 an estimated 925,000 deaths were caused by **heart attack**, stroke and related diseases.

Q: You mean, there are absolutely no symptoms?

A: Well . . . there are very few absolutes these days. What might be possible symptoms of high blood pressure vary from person to person, and they could be symptoms of other health problems as well. But . . . most doctors say that if you're having headaches, heart palpitations, a flushed face, blurry vision, nosebleeds, a tough time catching your breath after exertion, fatigue, a strong need to urinate often (especially during the night), **tinnitus** (a ringing or buzzing in the ears), **vertigo** (feelings that you or the world is spinning dizzily) or any combination of these—well, then check your blood pressure to see if that's the problem.

Q: Can high blood pressure be cured?

A: Well, yes and no. **Primary**, or **essential, hypertension** (85 to 95 percent of all cases) is the kind of high blood pressure that seems to happen, either because of heredity or other unknown or hard-to-find factors. This kind of hypertension doesn't have a cure, but it is controllable through various means and procedures that we'll talk about soon. Essential hypertension is a by-product of one or several glitches in the body's system of checks and balances that regulates pressure in the arteries.

Secondary hypertension occurs as an offshoot of some other condition, very often kidney disease. (The kidney, in terms of high blood pressure, can be either culprit or victim; that is, it can either be kidney problems that cause the high blood pressure or high blood pressure that causes kidney problems. Either way, the renal [kidney] system is among the first to be considered when hypertension is present.) By controlling or curing the basic problem, secondary hypertension may just disappear.

Q: What can happen to me if I leave my high blood pressure undetected and untreated?

A: You could find yourself being referred to in the past tense. Besides the aforementioned stroke, high blood pressure is a nicely paved highway leading to heart attack, **congestive heart failure**, **coronary-artery disease** and other high-speed exit ramps from this life. By making the heart work harder to push blood through the vascular system, high blood pressure—in the form of **hypertensive heart disease**—can make the heart grow in size and at the same time tire it out, with unhappy consequences. Further, it's believed that the increase in blood pressure eases the way for fatty deposits to build up on the artery walls and eventually clog them.

Studies have indicated that hypertension might also shrink the brain and may affect intellectual function. Surveying the literature on the subject, University of Pittsburgh researchers found that people with hypertension consistently scored lower than those with normal blood pressure on memory, attention and abstract reasoning tests. However, the researchers are unsure whether these impairments are caused by high blood pressure or are a by-product of the processes that trigger hypertension. And a study reported in the December 20, 1995, *Journal of the American Medical Association* found that the risk of poor cognitive function at midlife increased progressively with increasing levels of systolic pressure. For every increase of 10 mm Hg, the risk of poor cognitive function increased 9 percent.

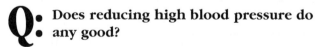

Q: **Does reducing high blood pressure do any good?**

A: Yes, reducing hypertension pays off in big ways. A study of 37,000 people, reported in *Lancet,* found that for every five to six points that a person's blood pressure is reduced, the risk of coronary heart disease declines by 20 to 25 percent and the risk of stroke by 30 to 40 percent.

Another study examined data from the Framingham Heart Study—the Cadillac of cardio-vascular risk factor reports—and the National Health and Nutritional Examination Survey II. The data suggest that reducing diastolic blood pressure by 2 mm Hg across the mean population through lifestyle modifications can greatly reduce the incidence of coronary heart disease and stroke. Specifically, this 2 mm Hg reduction would result in a 17 percent decrease in the prevalence of high blood pressure and a 6 percent reduction in risk of stroke, according to a study in *Archives of Internal Medicine.*

Q: **When the doctor tells me my high blood pressure is "benign" or "mild," does that mean I don't have anything to worry about?**

A: Not necessarily. What it means is that your hyper-tension isn't **accelerated**, or **malignant**, an extremely serious advanced stage of the disease.

But that doesn't mean you should dismiss your level of hypertension. As pointed out in the text-book *Principles of Internal Medicine,* "Hyper-tension is never truly benign, since even mild elevations of diastolic pressure are associated with increased risks of premature death and of vascular complications involving eyes, brain, heart and kidneys."

Just to be sure that you know what readings are considered problematic, let's review the current wisdom.

Category*	Systolic BP (mm Hg)	Diastolic BP (mm Hg)
Optimal	<120	<80
Normal	120-129	80-84
High normal	130-139	85-89
Hypertension		
Stage 1	140-159	90-99
Stage 2	160-179	100-109
Stage 3	180-209	110-119
Stage 4	≥210	≥120

*Based on an average of two or more readings on two or more occasions in individuals not taking antihypertensive medications and not acutely ill. When average falls in different categories of systolic and diastolic blood pressure, the higher category applies. Table based on recommendations of the Fifth Joint National Committee on Detection, Evaluation and Treatment of High Blood Pressure, National Heart, Lung and Blood Institute, National Institutes of Health.

Q: **What about white-coat hypertension, which we discussed previously? Does it require treatment?**

A: At the very least, your practitioner should keep an eye on it. For years the general agreement among medical professionals has been that white-coat hypertension is not associated with increased cardiovascular risk. However, a small Japanese study, reported in the journal *Hypertension*, found that people with white-coat hypertension and truly hypertensive people have similar enlargements of the left atrium and ventricle, compared with people with normal blood pressure. Some studies, too, have found that such changes precede more serious heart problems.

The question of whether a person with white-coat hypertension should be given drug treatment remains controversial, according to a *Lancet* article. Opinions differ about management; however, "the bulk of evidence suggests that drug treatment can be less aggressive than in patients whose pressure is persistently raised." (We'll talk more about antihypertensive medications later.)

Q: **Are men more likely than women to have high blood pressure?**

A: According to the AHA, men have a greater risk of high blood pressure than women until age 55. From age 55 to 75, the risks for men and women are about equal; after that, more women than men develop hypertension. Women's increasing risk of high blood pressure as they age, compared with men's, may be attributed to women outliving men, since many elderly people develop hypertension.

The latest figures from the AHA show that 20,090 women died from hypertension in 1991, versus 14,520 men.

Q: **Do women have any other special concerns regarding high blood pressure?**

A: Yes. And one of their concerns should be the exclusion of women in hypertension studies. Much of what is known about hypertension is the result of studies using male subjects exclusively.

Q: Why are researchers leaving out women?

A: Some medical experts say they have difficulty recruiting female participants or are hesitant to administer medication to pregnant women and women of childbearing age. Another reason may be that women younger than 55 don't have as high a risk as men; researchers tend to like to see results quickly, so they study higher-risk populations.

Q: What *is* known about women's particular concerns in regard to hypertension?

A: In a 1995 *Archives of Internal Medicine* article, Norman M. Kaplan, M.D., chief of the division of hypertension at the University of Texas Southwestern Medical Center in Dallas, summarized the following important points about women and hypertension:

- The latest figures available from the AHA show that 27 percent of women ages 18 to 74 have hypertension.

- Hypertension appears to cause less cardiovascular damage in women than it does in men. Researchers believe that estrogen, the hormone that controls the reproductive process in the female body, may play a role in minimizing damage from high blood pressure in women— although studies have not confirmed this hypothesis.

- Oral contraceptives, commonly called the Pill, usually cause a slight increase in blood pressure. In a small percentage of women, the rise is enough to induce hypertension. Smoking seems to further increase the risk.

- For women who have gone through menopause, the use of hormone replacement therapy almost never raises blood pressure and may decrease the risk of heart disease.

- Women benefit more from lifestyle modifications, such as improved diets and exercise programs, than do men.

- Studies show that high blood pressure in women responds to standard hypertension medication, although when death rates and complications are analyzed, women seem to derive less benefit from drug therapy.

Q: Are white Americans more likely than other ethnic-American groups to have high blood pressure?

A: No. According to AHA statistics, the opposite is true. African Americans, Puerto Ricans and Cuban- and Mexican-Americans are more likely to suffer from high blood pressure than Anglo-Americans.

Q: So it seems that an older African-American woman would have a high risk of developing hypertension. Right?

A: Right. In fact, according to the AHA figures, 39 percent of African-American women ages 18 to 74 have hypertension, compared with 25 percent of white women. The data suggest that the hypertensive African-American woman has a very high risk of renal failure, stroke or heart attack.

According to *Body & Soul: The Black Women's Guide to Physical Health and Emotional Well-Being,* this high rate of hypertension may be linked to lifestyle factors. Many of the foods of the traditional African-American diet are salty and fatty, dietary characteristics that may promote hypertension. The obesity rate within the black female population is also high—60 percent of black women between the ages of 45 and 75 are above the ideal body weight for their height, frame and age. The daily stresses that many black women face may be a contributing factor too.

Q: **Is blood pressure affected by the weather? By the changing seasons?**

A: As a matter of fact, it is—for certain people. If you have normal blood pressure, there's no seasonal variation. However, according to researchers at the Osaka University Medical School in Japan, people with essential hypertension can expect slightly higher blood pressure in winter than in summer. The reason given for this is complicated and merely educated guessing.

Q: **During a physical examination, my doctor looked in my eyes to see if I had high blood pressure. How come? What could he see?**

A: He did this because high blood pressure causes changes in the **retina**—from constriction of the

arterioles to more serious bleeding and optic damage. The retina is the only place in the human body where the arteries and arterioles can be looked at directly. And, as a result of a retinal examination, a medical practitioner can gain a lot of information about which stage of hypertension a person is in and what needs to be done. The worse the changes in the retina, the worse the prognosis.

Q: **Does blood pressure go up when you get older?**

A: We touched upon this earlier. Blood pressure often goes up as a person ages, but it doesn't have to. Research suggests that age-related increases in blood pressure are usually due to lifestyle factors, such as diet and frequency of exercise, rather than genetic influences. Three recent studies— in the United States, in Sweden and in the United Kingdom—provide evidence that management of blood pressure in the elderly markedly reduces incidence of **cardiovascular disease**.

The point here is that hypertension should not be viewed as an inevitable consequence of aging but should be taken into consideration, regardless of the age of the person whose systolic pressure edges up over 140 or whose diastolic pressure exceeds 90, according to an *Internal Medicine News & Cardiology News* article.

Q: Back to this business of rising blood pressure and the aging process. What's the story? Why does it go up so often?

A: When blood pressure rises as you get older, it's frequently related to **arteriosclerosis**—"hardening of the arteries"—which affects the elasticity of the arteries and the flow of blood through them, and which puts increased pressure on the more rigid vessel walls. Arteriosclerosis and **atherosclerosis**—the most prevalent form of arteriosclerosis and the major cause of stroke and heart attack in the United States—are trademarks of high blood pressure and a dizzying spiral to ill health, because not only does high blood pressure lead to the development and worsening of arteriosclerosis and atherosclerosis, but the worsening of these diseases then can lead to higher blood pressure readings.

On average, systolic blood pressure reaches an average value of 140 mm Hg by the time most Americans are in their 70s or 80s. In extreme cases, systolic pressure balloons up past 200 mm Hg in about one-tenth of all older folks. Diastolic pressure tends to increase with age but at a less steep rate than systolic pressure, and the value tends to remain constant or decline after the 50s.

Q: Can nervousness raise my blood pressure?

A: It can, especially if it's a long-term nervousness, or what is normally called psychological stress.

What happens, it seems, is that life's pressures cause the kidneys to retain sodium—but only if you're at high risk of developing high blood pressure in the first place (because of family history or a current high normal blood pressure). Combine this with a person's sympathetic nervous system tending to react in an exaggerated way to stress, and you've got a clear path ahead to blood pressure troubles.

Q: **Are you saying that emotions can influence blood pressure?**

A: Yes. While this is not a new idea, the first large prospective study on the topic just reported its findings in 1993. Researchers studied more than 1,000 men and women who completed a series of psychological questionnaires as part of the Framingham Heart Study and followed these people for 18 to 20 years. Among middle-aged men, those who developed hypertension had reported significantly higher levels of anxiety at the beginning of the study than those with normal blood pressure. Men who'd reported high levels of anxiety had more than twice the relative risk of developing hypertension than men who reported no anxiety.

Q: **What about the women in this study?**

A: Interestingly, levels of anxiety had no effect on the women's risk of hypertension.

Q: Back to stress—isn't it primarily a problem of the workplace?

A: Not at all. Home pressures, family problems, money problems, even excessive noise are all stressful situations that can lead to high blood pressure and cardiovascular disease. And even game-playing stresses can do it—blood pressure can rise like a guided missile while a person is playing a video game.

Q: If stress is the problem behind my high blood pressure, what can I do to unstress myself?

A: Your doctor might put you on antihypertensive medication and let it go at that, or perhaps urge you to exercise to work off your nervous energy.

On the other hand, certain kinds of behavioral therapies have been shown to work. Deep-breathing relaxation training, in combination with diet and sodium reduction, has allowed many people to go off their medication completely with no risk. **Biofeedback** is another technique of tuning in to the body's own calming rhythms that's met with success, as has progressive muscular relaxation.

Meditation is a well-known relaxer, and studies performed and reported by researchers employed by Maharishi International University—the think-tank arm of the Maharishi Maheshi Yogi's transcendental meditation movement—claim that meditators' systolic blood pressures are significantly lower than the blood pressures of same-age nonmeditators.

And studies show conclusively that owning a pet or merely watching fish swim in a tank can do wonders for your blood pressure health.

Behavioral therapists certainly can be recommended by your physician. The other forms of relaxation may not exactly be your doc's cup of tea. You can probably get a lead on these techniques, and others, by asking at your neighborhood Y or checking out the yellow pages.

The Chinese knew about behavioral therapy for high blood pressure long before the condition had a fancy medical name like hypertension. Ancient Chinese doctors recommended "placidity under all circumstances." It's a theory that works as well today as it did back then.

Q: Can people with high blood pressure exercise safely?

A: Not only can most high blood pressure sufferers exercise safely, but the exercise can bring their blood pressure down. You just shouldn't overdo, although a physical education instructor at the Pennsylvania State University has shown that hypertensives not on medication can exercise moderately—walking, jogging or swimming— even in temperatures up to 100°F. The exercise ought to have weight loss as its goal.

It's tough to say for sure if exercise alone lowers blood pressure. The drop could be the result of exercise-induced weight loss or a change in body sodium levels. But that's for scientists to argue over. Just so long as it does something good, it's worth the doing, even without knowing all the whys and wherefores.

Aerobic exercise benefits cases of mild and

moderate high blood pressure—or, in the language of the new classification system, stage 1 to stage 3 hypertension—but it's been kind of a no-no to do **isometric exercise**. The pushing, grunting and straining of the isometric resistance routines have been viewed traditionally as blood pressure elevators. However, newer studies are indicating that, yes, blood pressure might go up at the beginning, but the long-term effects are those of blood pressure reduction.

But before you start, have a long talk about an exercise regimen with somebody who knows—a qualified fitness instructor, for example.

Q: **You mean that even a simple walking routine can help?**

A: Definitely. Walking as infrequently as three times a week has been found to produce significant drops in resting diastolic blood pressure in some people. This is consistent with various reports that moderate aerobic activity is useful for managing mild (stage 1 to stage 2) primary hypertension.

Q: **Are there any exercises to absolutely avoid?**

A: We wouldn't recommend the marathon, at least not right off the bat. And the blood-pressure-raising strain associated with weight training is pretty much a no-no. Remember, moderation is the key.

One piece of equipment to avoid if you have moderate to high blood pressure (stage 3 and above) is the inversion bar and shoes, or anti-gravity boots, as they are sometimes called. What you do with this gear is simply hang upside down. It's supposed to be good for the spine and the body's musculature, and some aficionados love doing gut-ripping sit-ups and other calisthenics while dangling from the bar like a bat. Inversion therapy is bad news, however, even for healthy, nonhypertensive types. After only three minutes of this suspended inanimation, people with normal blood pressure have readings of 150/100.

Q: If I have high blood pressure, do I have to give up driving?

A: Probably not. The research into this area hasn't been able to pick up any real long- or short-term health hazards for the hypertensive. So, rev 'er up . . . but be sure to buckle up first.

Q: And how about sex?

A: Yeah, how about it! Sexual intercourse has a great elevating effect, not the least of which has to do with blood pressure. Systolic blood pressure levels can shoot up a whopping 107 percent, diastolic up as much as 60 percent, and heartbeat a'pounding up to 120 percent faster than usual. Some people have had coital blood pressures coming in at 300/175 mm Hg, or 237/138 on the mean for men and 216/127 for women. The peak is reached at orgasm; less than two minutes later, blood pressure has receded to levels lower than those before sex. Higher levels are hit when sex is had with a new or unfamiliar partner—opening night jitters, apparently.

Look, we can't tell you what to do—every case is different, and people have different needs and priorities. Some people can handle it, others are in real danger of going out in a blaze of glory. Your health-care professional can best answer your questions about how safe having sex is for you. Good luck.

Q: I'm a smoker. Should I stop if I have high blood pressure?

A: You should stop even if you don't have high blood pressure, but especially if you do. There's enough evidence to point an accusing finger at smoking as one of the major risk factors in the development of high blood pressure, and as a bad guy in accelerated cardiovascular disease.

Studies have shown that while no one knows for sure exactly how tobacco smoke causes vascular disease, it's pretty clear that smoking causes the body to release more **catecholamines** into the system. Catecholamines are chemicals the body produces in response to stress. They make the heart beat faster and with greater force, and cause blood vessels to constrict, among other things. This increase in **cardiac output** raises the blood pressure. Smoking speeds up release of the hormone **vasopressin**, and this too elevates blood pressure.

Researchers at the University of Southern California School of Medicine showed that if a person inhales nicotine-containing smoke, the production of **prostacyclin**—a chemical that dilates, or expands, the openings of blood vessels—is reduced. By doing so, nicotine smoke is directly involved in higher blood pressure and, perhaps, more extensive coronary heart damage.

And if that isn't enough to get you off your butt, yet another study, this from the cardiovascular center of New York Hospital-Cornell Medical Center, outlined a connection between smoking and blockage of the kidney's artery (**renal artery stenosis**, to use the technical terminology). What the scientists found was that of those who were suffering from renal artery stenosis, all had significantly higher systolic and diastolic blood pressures, and 94 percent of the men and 74 percent of the women were smokers.

Finally, yet another recent study showed that nearly three-fourths of women who had been hospitalized for malignant hypertension were smokers, oral contraceptive users or both.

What this says, clearly, is that if you discover you have high blood pressure, giving up smoking has got to be one of the first steps you take. Giving it up before developing the condition is better yet. Best of all is never smoking to begin with. An ounce of prevention is worth a pound of hypertension.

Q: Well, now that I know that smoking is bad for my blood pressure, what else do I have to look out for?

A: If you drink alcoholic beverages, you might want to reconsider the ways you wet your whistle.

Q: You mean you're going to take booze away from me, too?

A: No. You have to take it away from yourself. The evidence is fairly strong that those who tipple may topple.

When 4,783 men and women 20 years of age and older were studied by a team of scientists at the University of California at San Diego to see how drinking affected their blood pressure, the results (published in the journal *Hypertension*) indicated that as little as the equivalent of two stiff belts a day (30 milliliters of alcohol, or slightly less than an ounce) was all it took to produce a "modest but consistent" increase in both systolic and diastolic pressure readings. The researchers noted that men 35 years of age or older downing that amount of booze were nearly twice as likely to have high blood pressure as nondrinkers. And the direct correlation is clear: Blood pressure was especially high if those examined had had alcohol during the previous 24 hours.

According to a doctor working with the Stanford Heart Disease Prevention Program, by increasing alcohol consumption from one to three drinks per day in men 50 to 74 years old, systolic pressure would rise just as much as if the body weight of those men had increased from 165 to 195 pounds. He also offered the theory that if you have at least one or two drinks a day, and if you also have high blood pressure and you're over 50, you should try abstaining for a while—your blood pressure could go down, thus saving you all kinds of doctors' bills and unnecessary medication costs and side effects.

Exactly how and why alcohol affects blood pressure isn't known—it just does. And that's important to know.

Q: How do my eating habits affect my blood pressure?

A: What you eat—and how much—has a lot to do with where your blood pressure level resides.

As a general rule, obesity and high blood pressure go hand-in-pudgy-hand. Obesity may cause high blood pressure which in turn may cause cardiovascular disease, but—as with nearly everything in the study of blood pressure—the mechanism is not clear. In fact, it may not be there at all. Obesity and high blood pressure could be totally independent problems, merely existing side by side in the body of a person with heart disease. While many scientific studies show that the blood pressure of certain overweight people drops when those people drop some poundage, other studies have indicated that the hypertensive obese person may not be in any greater danger of heart attack and heart-related deaths than a nonobese hypertensive—and, in fact, the obese person may be in less danger. Others say that weight loss without antihypertensive drug therapy at the same time may have no real and lasting effect on individuals with mild (stage 1 to stage 2) hypertension.

Still and all, it probably pays to lose weight, whether or not it shows up immediately on your blood pressure scorecard. Besides looking and feeling better, you probably will live longer too. According to the Society of Actuaries, if you are 30 percent above average weight, your risk of dying from coronary disease, compared with people of average weight, is 44 percent higher for men and 34 percent higher for women. Whether that has to do with blood pressure is moot—and irrelevant, really. It has to do with living, and that should be sufficient motivation.

Q: **Are there any specific foods to stay away from?**

A: Well, you might want to at least cut down on coffee and meat, if not cut them out entirely.

For years debate has ensued on whether coffee, or caffeine intake, has an elevating effect on blood pressure. Early studies from Duke University and Harvard Medical School said it was a sure thing. The Duke study, especially, drew a clear connection between caffeine, high blood pressure and stress; it showed that a few cups of coffee can raise blood pressure, and when work-related stress or everyday pressures were factored in, the mixture wasn't good, especially for java-gulping, tense office workers. Wrote the Duke researcher in an issue of *Psychosomatic Medicine*: "Blood pressure increases of the magnitude seen in the present study could potentially eliminate or reverse the therapeutic effects of a number of the antihypertensive medications currently in use."

A more recent study—this one of more than 45,000 men by researchers at Harvard University School of Public Health—exonerated coffee as a heart risk factor. The researchers reported in the *New England Journal of Medicine* that men who drank even as much as four cups of coffee a day had no higher risk of developing heart disease than those men who drank no coffee at all. For some folks, then, a moderate amount of coffee, but not an excess, might be okay. For you? You might want to try it both ways—with coffee and without—and see how your blood pressure reacts.

As for meat eating, it too has been linked to increased blood pressure. A few studies demonstrating that connection may have been tainted because they looked at how vegetarians (who often have better blood pressure readings than omnivores) reacted to meat—never thinking that part of the observed blood pressure rise was the result of anxiety of nonmeat-eaters eating the stuff. However, at least one newer study took "regular" meat-eaters, put them on a veggie diet, watched as blood pressures dropped, put them back on their usual meals and saw their blood pressures go back up again.

You needn't feel obliged to become a total vegetarian, but cutting down on meat is probably a good idea.

Q: Anything else?

A: Uh-huh. Cut down on fats. When you need to use them, use the monounsaturated, such as olive oil and canola oil. Or use the polyunsaturated kind, such as corn, safflower, sunflower, cottonseed, soybean and walnut oils, which may have a **diuretic** effect.

Q: I've heard conflicting reports about margarine and butter. Which one should I be using?

A: The confusion began when trans fatty acids—formed when liquid polyunsaturated vegetable oils are processed to make solid or semisolid margarine—were thought to be better for you than saturated fats such as butter. But further research indicated that trans fatty acids act in ways similar to saturated fats—both seem to aggravate the risk factors of hypertension and other heart conditions. "While the link [between margarine and heart disease] has not yet been proven beyond a reasonable doubt, it would be prudent to lower the amount of margarines and trans fatty acids in the diet and switch to mono-unsaturated fats such as olive oil," said a leading researcher in *Circulation.*

In short, the current advice (but who's to say when the next shift in thinking will take place and where the shift will take us) for those who insist on including margarine in their diets is to stick with soft-spread margarines, which have fewer trans fatty acids per gram than stick margarines. Look for those that list water or a liquid vegetable oil as the first ingredient. If you've been melting margarine to use in cooking, switch to olive or canola oil instead.

Q: Isn't there some sort of fat in fish that's supposed to be good for your blood pressure?

A: Maybe or maybe not. Some fatty fish, such as salmon, mackerel, tuna and some shellfish, contain omega-3 fatty acids and have been heralded to have a beneficial effect on blood pressure and cardiac health in general. However, a large 1995 Harvard study, reported in the *New England Journal of Medicine,* found contradictory results. In this study, men whose diets were richest in omega-3 fatty acids had a slightly higher risk of coronary disease (12 percent) and underwent more coronary bypass operations than those whose diets were lowest in omega-3 fatty acids. But to complicate matters, the same study found that men who ate any amount of fish, as opposed to men who didn't, had a 26 percent lower risk of contracting coronary disease. This finding led researchers to conclude that any benefits of omega-3 do not increase with increased intake.

In the November 1, 1995, issue of the *Journal of the American Medical Association,* a study found that eating one fatty fish meal a week was associated with a 50 percent reduction in the risk of cardiac arrest.

Q: What's the medical wisdom concerning dietary fiber?

A: You should increase your intake. The following foods are high in dietary fiber:

Food High in Dietary Fiber

Food	Portion Size	Grams of Fiber
100% bran cereal	1 cup	19.9
Baked beans	½ cup	8.3
Apple	1 medium	7.9
Broccoli, cooked stalk	1 medium	7.4
Spinach, cooked	½ cup	5.7
Almonds	¼ cup	5.1
Kidney beans	½ cup	4.5
Cabbage, shredded, boiled	½ cup	4.3
Shredded wheat	1 cup	4.3
Peas, cooked	½ cup	4.2
White beans	½ cup	4.2
Banana	1 medium	4.0
Corn	½ cup	3.9
Potato	1 medium	3.9
Pear	1 medium	3.8
Lentils	½ cup	3.7
Lima beans, cooked	½ cup	3.5
Sweet potato	1 medium	3.5
Pinto beans	½ cup	3.1
Peanuts, chopped	¼ cup	2.9
Brown rice, raw	¼ cup	2.8
Cornflakes	1 cup	2.8
Oats, rolled	½ cup	2.8
Orange	1 medium	2.6
Raisins	¼ cup	2.5
Brussels sprouts	4	2.4
Peanut butter	2 tablespoons	2.4
Whole wheat bread	1 slice	2.4
Apricots	3 medium	2.3
Carrots, raw	1 medium	2.3
Beets	½ cup	2.1

(continued on following page)

Food High in Dietary Fiber, *continued*

Food	Portion Size	Grams of Fiber
Peaches	1 medium	2.1
Kale, cooked	½ cup	2.0
Zucchini, raw	½ cup	2.0

Sources: Adapted from

McCance and Widdowson's *The Composition of Foods,* by
A. A. Paul and D. A. T. Southgate (Elsevier/North-Holland
Biomedical, 1978).

Nutritive Value of American Foods in Common Units,
Agriculture Handbook 456 (U.S. Department of Agriculture,
1975).

"Composition of Foods Commonly Used in Diets for Persons
With Diabetes," by James W. Anderson, Wen-Ju Lin and
Kyleen Ward, *Diabetes Care,* September/October 1978.

Composition of Foods: Soups, Sauces and Gravies, Agriculture
Handbook 8-6 (U.S. Department of Agriculture, 1980).

Composition of Foods: Spices and Herbs, Agriculture
Handbook 8-6 (U.S. Department of Agriculture, 1980).

"Topics in Dietary Fiber" and "Fiber Analysis Tables,"
Reports of Research of the Cornell University Agricultural
Experiment Station, 1978.

Information supplied by cereal companies.

Q: And what about salt? That's supposed to be bad for me, isn't it?

A: Well, as we've been seeing, nothing's easy to say for sure when it comes to blood pressure. And the subject of salt in the diet is another uncertainty that's grown into a full-blown controversy—one that's been brewing for nearly 80 years of blood pressure research.

To start off with, the mineral sodium is necessary for human well-being. Sodium is a part of many foods and food additives. Salt is 40 percent sodium, and salt is the vehicle by which most of us get our daily portion of sodium. The problem is this: Our daily portion is just too high. We only need 200 milligrams a day, but most of us are sopping up as much as 30 times that amount.

True, most of us don't have any adverse reaction to sodium. However, it's likely that there are some people who are genetically programmed to react to sodium by having their blood pressure rise.

If we have learned anything in this book, it is that nobody knows for sure the mechanism for anything that has to do with blood pressure—and the sodium/high-blood-pressure connection is no exception. Some scientists believe that blood pressure goes up in the people in which it does go up because sodium increases water retention, and the result is greater arterial pressure. But that's just conjecture at the moment.

There's no real controversy about salt/sodium in some way causing high blood pressure in people genetically susceptible to sodium's effects. The brouhaha has to do with the idea that by cutting back on sodium via low-salt diets, all Americans can avoid getting high blood pressure. There is no clear evidence that that is actually the case.

In other words, salt will more than likely raise your blood pressure if you already have high blood pressure (although this won't happen in all hypertensive people), but it won't necessarily raise your blood pressure if you're **normotensive** (have blood pressure in the normal range).

Q: So that settles it, huh? Salt's not so bad after all?

A: Remember, in Bloodpressureland, nothing is ever settled . . . except, perhaps, estates. Everybody's got a theory, and the guns on one side are as big and respectable as those on the other. Take, for example, this quote from the chancellor of the University of Tennessee Center for Health Sciences: "In the absence of proved need or benefit and because of the potential harm, excessive sodium consumption by the American public is justified cause for concern." Or here's one from the chairman of the department of physiology at the University of Maryland School of Medicine, who calls the sodium/high-blood-pressure link "dangerously minimized."

Or look at the research from a study conducted in the Netherlands that involved newborn babies. Half of the group of infants were put on a normal-sodium diet for the first six months of their lives, while the rest of the kids ate a low-sodium menu. Results: The normal-sodium babies developed higher blood pressure than the lower-sodium group, leading the doctors conducting the study to conclude that blood pressure is related to sodium intake, and that "moderation of sodium intake, starting very early in life, might perhaps contribute to prevention of high blood pressure and of rise of blood pressure with age."

On the other hand, some experts maintain that other factors cloud the issue: the stresses of modern life, a host of other foods taken in too large or too small amounts, lack of exercise and so on.

Q: Hasn't any study isolated these various factors?

A: So glad you asked. One recent landmark study did indeed isolate the salt/high-blood-pressure link, putting to rest some of the concerns about other factors influencing test results. In the Australian study, reported in the journal *Nature Medicine,* researchers found that adding salt to chimpanzees' diets sent their blood pressure up significantly. When salt was removed, blood pressure came back down.

The lead researcher chose chimpanzees as subjects because the animal species is by far the closest biologically to humans. The particular chimpanzees he chose were living comfortably on a diet of mostly fruits and vegetables, in a long-established group, and were adjusted to the stresses in their lives. The addition of salt to their diet involved no other change.

While the study shows a direct link between dietary salt and high blood pressure, the researchers emphasize that high blood pressure in humans is complex. The influence of dietary salt is not as easily isolated in humans.

Q: So who's right and who's wrong?

A: Possibly everybody's a little right and perhaps everybody's a little wrong . . . maybe.

Q: It's all so confusing! What's a person to do?

A: A concerned person will be careful, not overdo, and eat smartly. The person with high blood pressure will go on a low-salt diet and see if that helps. It could help so much that further therapies, including antihypertensive drugs, will not be necessary, especially if yours is a mild (stage 1

to stage 2) hypertension, and you couple salt/
sodium reduction with weight loss.

The person with normal blood pressure will
control the urge to salt everything—just in case.
Besides, food tastes better without the salt. It
tastes like itself. That's not to say you should
abstain or put yourself through the hell of a bland
diet. A low-low-salt diet is not only frustrating—
eating tasty food is one of life's great pleasures—
but it also ensures the urge to cheat, indulge,
binge and, perhaps, pay the consequences . . .
whatever they may be. Listen to your body; heed
what it says to you; act—and eat—accordingly.

Q: Besides keeping the salt shaker off my
table, what else can I do to restrict the
sodium in my diet?

A: Here's what:

- Watch for the "hidden" sodium in canned,
  frozen or otherwise processed foods. Canned
  vegetables often have salt added to them. Even
  canned fruits may have salt in them.

- Don't go to all the trouble of keeping the
  shaker invisible while dining—then go and add
  salt to soups, stews, etc., while cooking. It does
  the same damage (that is, if it does damage).
  And make sure the same goes for when you eat
  out. All your willpower at the table can be for
  naught if the chef is going hog-wild with the
  salt in the kitchen, or is using flour with high
  sodium content, along with sodium-laden
  baking powder and baking soda. And if you're
  in a Chinese restaurant, be aware that the food
  is often liberally spiced with monosodium

glutamate (MSG), and this popular flavor enhancer has a high sodium content. Furthermore, don't add soy sauce or tamari to the food—both have lots of sodium and "hidden" MSG in them.

- Certain antacids are high in sodium, although in recent years new lines of antacids have been developed that are lower in sodium than their older cousins. Always check the label.

- Naturally occurring sodium can slip into your tum unbeknownst to even the most scrupulous dietitians. One of the sneakiest is milk (120 milligrams per cup). Celery, artichokes and spinach have moderate amounts of sodium too.

- Some drinking water may have a lot of natural sodium in it, but studies are inconclusive when it comes to whether it raises your blood pressure significantly.

- Be sure you understand the language of low-salt. In Food and Drug Administration-specified terms:
  —*Sodium-free* means less than 5 milligrams of sodium per serving.
  —*Very low sodium* means 35 milligrams or less per serving.
  —*Low sodium* means 140 milligrams or less per serving.
  —*Reduced sodium* means the usual level of sodium has been cut by at least 25 percent.
  —*Unsalted, no salt added* or some equivalent phrase refers to food once processed with salt but now produced without it—although the food may contain other forms of sodium.

- Become expert at fixing your meals with spices that will make you forget that there is even anything called sodium. For example:

—On eggs, try dill, oregano or chopped chives, individually or mixed together.

—For mashed potatoes, boil the potatoes with a clove of garlic, mash the potatoes, add chopped parsley, cayenne pepper, paprika, dill or curry powder.

—Season vegetables with nutmeg.

—Rub chicken with garlic, sprinkle with lemon juice and dust with paprika, sage and thyme.

—Rub red meats with fresh ginger and add rosemary or crushed black pepper.

—Dump out the salt and fill the shakers with oregano, basil, thyme, caraway seeds, sesame seeds or poppy seeds.

—Other spices to experiment with are allspice, chili powder, curry, ground mustard, peppermint, tarragon, coriander, cardamom, cumin, cloves and celery seeds.

Q: Any other things good for me to eat for my high blood pressure?

A: Besides what's been discussed already, there are three major pieces of dietary advice: calcium, magnesium and potassium. Foods rich in these three minerals—and high in their ratio to sodium—are generally conceded to be blood pressure lowerers and heart protectors.

Let's take calcium first. Results of a Cornell University Medical College study point to the importance of calcium in the workings and the therapy of hypertension. Other research—and there is a good deal of it—has shown that hypertensive people eat less calcium than normotensive people; that when as many as 17 different nutrients were examined, it was only the calcium level that separated the high blood pressure sufferers from those with normal blood pressure; that a group of people without high blood pressure who added one gram (1,000 milligrams) of calcium to their daily diets had drops in their diastolic blood pressures; and that some scientists think that the way doctor-prescribed diuretics lower blood pressure is by increasing serum calcium levels. The evidence that calcium is an antihypertensive, when taken at daily levels of about 1,000 to 1,500 milligrams, is pretty convincing.

Here is a chart showing foods high in calcium that are also low in sodium:

Foods High in Calcium
(And Low in Sodium)

Food	Portion Size	Calcium (mg)	Sodium (mg)
Swiss cheese	2 ounces	544	148
Yogurt (skim milk)	1 cup	452	174
Yogurt (low-fat)	1 cup	415	159
Milk, skim	1 cup	302	126
Milk, low-fat	1 cup	297	122
Tofu	4 ounces	145	8
Blackstrap molasses	1 tablespoon	137	19
Collards, cooked	½ cup	110	18
Kale, cooked	½ cup	103	24
Mustard greens	½ cup	97	13
Watercress (chopped)	½ cup	95	33
Almonds	¼ cup	83	1.5
Salmon, fresh	4 ounces	79	60
Chickpeas, dried	¼ cup	75	13
Broccoli	½ cup	68	8

Sources: USDA Handbooks 8, 8-1 and 456; U.S. Department of Agriculture Nutrient Data Research Group, 1983.

Q: And magnesium? Is that as effective as calcium?

A: Yes. Study after study from all over the world shows that daily doses of magnesium, either through supplementation or in the diet, can keep blood pressure in its place.

The accompanying list offers most good food sources of magnesium. But, depending on your diet, you might feel that you need a supplement to be certain of getting at least the recommended dietary allowance of 350 milligrams a day for

Foods High in Magnesium

Food	Portion Size	Magnesium (mg)
Soy flour, full fat	½ cup	180
Tofu (soybean curd), raw	½ cup	127
Almonds, unblanched	¼ cup	105
Black-eyed peas, dried	¼ cup	98
Soybeans, dry	¼ cup	98
Wheat germ, toasted	¼ cup	91
Cashews	¼ cup	89
Brazil nuts, unblanched	¼ cup	79
Swiss chard, cooked	½ cup	75
Rye flour	½ cup	74
Whole wheat flour	½ cup	68
Peanuts, dry-roasted	¼ cup	64
Walnuts, black	¼ cup	63
Peanut flour, defatted	¼ cup	56
Oatmeal	1 cup	56
Shredded wheat	1 cup	55
Potato, baked	1 medium	55

(continued on opposite page)

men, 300 milligrams for women. And, if so, keep in mind that magnesium works best when accompanied by about two times as much calcium. Also be alerted to the fact that so-called soft water has fewer minerals in it than the "hard" kind—and magnesium is among the missing. If your drinking water supply is "soft" or softened, you might want supplementation all the more—because of the process involved, sodium levels are elevated in softened water, and studies show greater amount of heart disease among soft water-imbibing communities.

Food	Portion Size	Magnesium (mg)
Blackstrap molasses	1 tablespoon	52
Beet greens, cooked	½ cup	49
Lima beans, baby, boiled	¼ cup	49
Spinach, raw, chopped	1 cup	44
Salmon, sockeye, canned	4 ounces	44
Kidney beans, boiled	½ cup	40
Avocado	½	40
Banana	1 medium	35
Pecans, halved	¼ cup	35
Milk, skim	1 cup	28
Brown rice	½ cup	28
Peanut butter	1 tablespoon	25
Beef, round, lean	3 ounces	24
Buckwheat flour, light	½ cup	24
Chestnuts, roasted	½ cup	24
Collards, cooked	1 cup	22

Source: *The Complete Book of Vitamins and Minerals for Health* (Rodale Press, 1988).

Q: And potassium?

A: Same story. Diets high in potassium seem to aid in the reduction of high blood pressure, particularly hypertension that's also connected with sodium intake. Israeli scientists announced, after a goodly amount of research, that they felt that it was potassium that was the key antihypertensive agent in the vegetarian diet.

There are various theories as to how potassium works in keeping blood pressure down; nobody knows for sure, but it's felt that it acts as a diuretic, moving excess water from the blood vessel cell walls. In this way, it's an antagonist of sodium, which works hard as a water retainer. So lots of food scientists believe that foods high in potassium and low in sodium are crucial for blood pressure control.

Here's a list of foods with a high potassium-to-sodium ratio, along with a list that's vice versa. Note that canned and frozen foods aren't on the first list; that's because the canning and freezing processes change the potassium-sodium ratio in a negative way. For some eye-opening examples, see the list of processed foods.

Foods High in Potassium
(And Low in Sodium)

Food	Portion Size	Potassium (mg)	Sodium (mg)
Fresh vegetables			
Asparagus	½ cup	165	1
Avocado	½	680	5
Carrot, raw	1	225	38
Corn	½ cup	136	trace
Lima beans, cooked	½ cup	581	1
Potato	1 medium	782	6
Spinach, cooked	½ cup	292	45
Squash, winter	½ cup	473	1
Tomato, raw	1 medium	444	5
Fresh fruits			
Apple	1 medium	182	2
Apricots, dried	¼ cup	318	9
Banana	1 medium	440	1
Cantaloupe	¼ melon	341	17
Orange	1 medium	263	1
Peach	1 medium	308	2
Plums	5	150	1
Strawberries	½ cup	122	trace
Unprocessed meats			
Chicken, light meat	3 ounces	350	54
Lamb, leg	3 ounces	241	53
Roast beef	3 ounces	224	49
Pork	3 ounces	219	48
Fish			
Cod	3 ounces	345	93
Flounder	3 ounces	498	201
Haddock	3 ounces	297	150
Salmon	3 ounces	378	99
Tuna, drained solids	3 ounces	225	38

Sources: USDA Handbooks 456 and 8-1.

Foods High in Sodium
(And Low in Potassium)

Food	Portion Size	Potassium (mg)	Sodium (mg)
Salt	1 teaspoon	trace	2,132
Soy sauce	1 teaspoon	22	1,123
Bouillon cube	1	4	960
Hard cheeses			
Parmesan	2 ounces	53	1,056
American	2 ounces	93	812
Brie	2 ounces	87	356
Muenster	2 ounces	77	356
Cheddar	2 ounces	56	352
Colby	2 ounces	72	342
Swiss	2 ounces	64	148
Cottage cheese (2% fat)	½ cup	110	561
Snack foods			
Pretzels, thin, twisted	10	10	1,008
Saltines	10	34	312
Potato chips	10	226	200
Peanuts, roasted salted	¼ cup	243	151
Processed meats			
Salami	3 ounces	170	1,043
Bologna	3 ounces	133	981
Frankfurter	3 ounces	136	1,003
Canned soups			
Chicken noodle	1 cup	53	1,049
Cream of mushroom (prepared with water)	1 cup	94	967
Tomato	1 cup	247	816
Vegetable beef	1 cup	162	896
Canned vegetables			
Beets	½ cup	142	200
Corn	½ cup	80	195
Lima beans	½ cup	188	200
Peas	½ cup	82	200

Sources: USDA Handbooks 456 and 8-1.

The preparation of foods is crucial to the potassium-sodium ratio. For example, the potato is normally a good source of potassium—but when boiled, as much as 50 percent of it floats away... and when boiled in salt water, nearly half the sodium in the water seeps into the potato. Bye-bye, positive ratio.

Here's a look at various cooking preparations of a potato—and their results. As you can see, steaming is the hands-down winner.

State of potatoes	Na+ (sodium) (mmol/l)	K+ (potassium) (mmol/l)	K+/Na+ (ratio)
Raw	1	104	104
Boiled (peeled) in 1% salt	90	64	0.7
Boiled (peeled) unsalted	1	79	79
Boiled (unpeeled) in 1% salt	30	84	2.8
Boiled (unpeeled) unsalted	1	94	94
Steamed (peeled) unsalted	1	100	100

The Difference Processing Can Make

	Portion Size	Potassium (mg)	Sodium (mg)
Menu I			
Roast beef	3 ounces	224	49
Potato, baked	1 medium	782	3
String beans, fresh	½ cup	95	2.5
Whole wheat bread, firm crumb	1 slice	68	132
Unsalted butter	1 tablespoon	4	1.4
Peaches, fresh sliced	½ cup	172	1
Milk, whole	1 cup	370	122
		1,715	310.9
Menu II			
Corned beef	3 ounces	51	802
Potatoes, hash brown, frozen	1 cup	439	463
String beans, canned	½ cup	64	159.5
White bread, soft crumb	1 slice	29	142
Butter	1 tablespoon	3	140
Peach pie	⅛ pie	176	316
Milk, whole	1 cup	370	122
		1,132	2,144.5

Sources: USDA Handbooks 456 and 8-1.

Q: I just found out that I have high blood pressure. What type of treatment is my doctor going to prescribe?

A: Your doctor's specific recommendations will depend on the degree of your hypertension and the state of your overall health.

Generally, there's one thing about blood pressure drug therapy that's important to remember:

Many health organizations recommend and many doctors practice a **stepped care** approach. This program suggests a series of progressively aggressive treatment options.

In the past, the steps of this course of treatment were well-defined with little variance among individual cases. However, the latest federal guidelines spelled out in the fifth report of the Joint National Committee on Detection, Evaluation and Treatment of High Blood Pressure (of the National Heart, Lung and Blood Institute, National Institutes of Health), popularly known as JNC-V, suggest that physicians carefully weigh treatment options, taking into consideration many factors, including the patient's age, race and presence of other disorders, rather than automatically prescribing the next step up in the ascending staircase.

Q: Okay, so what's the goal of treatment, and what's the first step?

A: The objective is to reduce morbidity and mortality by reducing and maintaining a blood pressure level below 140/90. And the first step—lifestyle modifications. We've mentioned these before: weight reduction, moderation of alcohol intake, regular exercise, reduction of sodium intake and smoking cessation.

Q: And if my blood pressure doesn't respond to my change in health habits, what's next?

A: You should continue your lifestyle modifications, and your practitioner will probably recommend a first-line antihypertensive medication. At times, lifestyle modifications are prescribed in conjunction with an antihypertensive medication right from the start.

Q: What kind of medication are we talking about?

A: The answer is complex. In the past, unless blood pressure was dangerously high and immediate reduction was a matter of life or death, the first type of drug most often prescribed by physicians was the diuretic.

Diuretics promote frequent urination—it's no mystery, then, why many people refer to them as water pills—which increases the elimination of water and sodium from the body, and decreases the blood volume, among other things. The diuretics most often prescribed are members of the **thiazide** family—Diuril, Dyazide and Corzide are a few of the many popular brand names—except for so-called loop diuretics, such as furosemide (Lasix) and bumetanide (Bumex), which are used for high blood pressure cases related to kidney disease.

Although once the most popular antihypertensives, today diuretics are not always given as the first-line therapy for high blood pressure. More and more physicians seem to prefer the newer, more expensive drugs: **angiotensin converting enzyme (ACE) inhibitors** (Capoten, Vasotec, etc.) and **calcium channel blockers** (Procardia, Cardizem, etc.).

Q: Why the switch?

A: That's where the controversy begins. Some physicians say they've started to prescribe these other medications as first-line therapy because of the side effects associated with diuretics (although it would do well for us to remember that all blood pressure medications have side effects).

The most frequent unwanted results of diuretic therapy are potassium and magnesium deficiency, gout and a possible rise in levels of cholesterol. The potassium and magnesium problems may be overcome by taking supplements in doses recommended by the physician. The gout is treated with yet another drug. And the cholesterol problem is usually helped by sticking to a low-fat diet.

Some experts also cite male sexual dysfunction as another adverse effect. There have also been studies indicating that diuretics increase the risk of cardiac arrest.

Q: So what's the controversy?

A: Well, not all medical experts believe the trend away from diuretics is related to the side effects. Instead, they insist it has more to do with the promotion of ACE inhibitors and other new agents by pharmaceutical companies. These new drugs, they say, are overshadowing the older options, such as diuretics and **beta-adrenergic blocking drugs** (or **beta blockers**), which are no longer marketed aggressively.

Q: Do you mean heavy duty marketing by drug manufacturers can make a difference in doctors' prescribing habits—for good or bad?

A: Yes.

Q: Isn't there an official opinion on the matter of first-line drug treatment?

A: The authors of the JNC-V, attempting to resolve the debate but instead refueling it, recently reemphasized their support of diuretics and beta blockers, as the *preferred* first-line therapy—if there are no contraindications or compelling reasons to choose another drug. However, their list of first-line therapies includes calcium channel blockers, ACE inhibitors and another drug, which we have not mentioned yet, **alpha-adrenergic blocking drugs**, or **alpha blockers** (Cardura, Minipress, etc.).

Q: Has any other group of note joined the fray?

A: Yes. In mid-1995 cardiologists at the annual meeting of the American Society of Hypertension agreed that diuretics may be underused by some physicians and that some groups of hypertensive people—the elderly and African Americans, in particular—benefit most from diuretic therapy.

Q: So what am I to believe and do?

A: We can't tell you what to believe, when even the experts disagree on the "facts." But we can suggest what you can do: Discuss the options with your doctor.

Q: You said that the JNC-V recommends diuretics and beta blockers as preferred first-line therapy. You've already told me how diuretics work. Can you now tell me how beta blockers lower hypertension?

A: Beta blockers reduce high blood pressure by reducing the force and speed of the heartbeat. Whereas diuretics affect blood pressure through indirect means—by reducing sodium, water and blood volume—beta blockers act directly on the heart, blood vessels and sympathetic nervous system. Beta blockers include propranolol (Inderal is the popular brand name version), nadolol (Corgard) and metoprolol (Lopressor).

Q: What about side effects?

A: Beta blockers may cause side effects. Common side effects include fatigue, slow heart rate, light-headedness, dizziness, insomnia, indigestion, nausea, vomiting and cold extremities. More serious, less common side effects include disorientation, depression, anxiety, decrease in libido, impotence, chest pains, impaired circulation and congestive heart failure (in persons with advanced heart disease).

Q: **What about the increasingly popular ACE inhibitors and calcium channel blockers? How do they work?**

A: ACE inhibitors block the production of angiotensin, a chemical the body produces to raise blood pressure. Angiotensin's normal role is to maintain equilibrium when blood pressure drops, by tightening the arteries. ACE inhibitors can bring pressure down quickly but can cause, although rarely, a reduction in the number of white blood cells, which leads to an increased susceptibility to infection. ACE inhibitors include captopril (Capoten), lisinopril (Prinivil, Zestril) and enalapril (Vasotec).

Calcium channel blockers work by blocking the passage of calcium, which the muscle cells use to control the size of the blood vessels. When the muscles of the arteries are prevented from constricting, blood vessels open up, allowing blood to flow more easily through them. Included in this class of drugs are nifedipine (Procardia), diltiazem (Cardizem), isradipine (DynaCirc) and verapamil (Calan). The common side effects are similar to those of beta blockers.

Q: Anything else to know?

A: Yes, and the news is not very good. Medical experts are currently debating the safety of certain calcium channel blockers due to their possible link to heart attacks. In an ongoing study of hypertensive people, reported in a 1995 issue of the *Journal of the American Medical Association,* the use of short-acting calcium channel blockers, especially in high doses, was associated with a 60 percent increase in risk for heart attacks.

In September 1995 the National Institutes of Health issued a warning that stated that short-acting nifedipine should be used "with great caution, if at all" and that the safety of related drugs was unclear.

Currently a study is in progress that will compare the use of various blood pressure drugs in 40,000 Americans. It is expected to provide a definitive assessment of the risks of calcium channel blockers—but won't be completed until 2002.

As with any prescribed medicine, discuss with your practitioner any acute or chronic conditions you may have before beginning treatment.

Q: There's one more drug on the first-line therapy list that you haven't explained. How do alpha blockers work?

A: These drugs work by blocking the nerve receptors called alpha receptors. Alpha receptors normally promote constriction of the arterioles. Blocking constriction promotes dilation of vessels and lowers blood pressure, as well as reduces the work of the heart in some situations. These drugs also inhibit the production and the effect of adrenaline, a potent stimulator released by the body in response to stress. Too much adrenaline can overexcite the circulatory system and cause blood pressure to climb.

Q: **What are the side effects of alpha blockers?**

A: The possible side effects include dizziness, fainting, nausea, headache and palpitations.

Q: **What if my blood pressure fails to respond to first-line drug therapy? What's the next step?**

A: That depends on your individual case. At one time, practitioners would begin with the mildest of drugs at the smallest of doses, then gradually increase the dosage of that drug to its maximum. Then if necessary, another stronger drug would be introduced at its mildest dosage. However, as we said earlier, practitioners have gotten away from this structured approach in favor of individualized care, and current guidelines don't necessarily dictate that a stronger drug is needed at this point. Your practitioner may suggest an increased dosage of your current medication or she may substitute another drug from the same or different drug class or add a second medication to your treatment program.

Q: Are there any other antihypertensive medications that we haven't talked about yet?

A: Yes. During the treatment of your high blood pressure you may hear of another class of drugs called **peripheral adrenergic antagonists**. Included in this class is reserpine (Serpasil).

Q: How does this class of drugs work?

A: Drugs in this class, which are among some of the older hypertensive medications, inhibit the release of or block the effect of adrenaline. This results in dilation of the blood vessels, allowing blood to flow easily. The major drawback of these medications is their sedating effect.

Q: Any others?

A: Yes. There are additional drugs that lower blood pressure by dilating the arteries. These strong **peripheral vasodilators** act directly on the muscles that comprise the walls of the artery, causing them to dilate. (ACE inhibitors, calcium channel blockers and alpha blockers are also peripheral vasodilators, but, as we've mentioned, they dilate the vessels indirectly.)

Some of the stronger vasodilators produce a very rapid reduction in blood pressure—especially when given by injection—and, therefore, are often used in a hypertensive crisis. The most common side effects include nausea and vomiting, headaches, dizziness and irregular heartbeat. Hydralazine (Apresoline) is included in this class.

Q: **Drug therapy seems to have been the turning point in the control of high blood pressure and the saving of lives. Right?**

A: There's no question that the discovery and availability of many prescription antihypertensive medications are the reasons a lot of us are up and about today. They have played critical, life-or-death roles in the human dramas of many sick people. But they should not be placed on a pedestal or given a godlike reverence. In fact, according American Heart Association statistics, high blood pressure deaths have markedly declined since 1940—and that's long before these drugs were even being dispensed. They are not *the* answer, just an answer, and maybe only the current answer . . . tools to be used when the machinery calls for it. And lately they're tools that continue to cause controversy within the medical community.

Q: **Really? Is there something wrong with them?**

A: Well, beyond the very evident side effects involved with the taking of many of these drugs—side effects that may outweigh the benefits of the medication—and the debate that we previously mentioned about first-line therapy, there is some very serious discussion going on about how long to take medicine for hypertension, and if there are long-lasting negatives associated with antihypertensive drug use.

Q: For instance . . . ?

A: For instance, the idea that's long circulated among medical practitioners that once you go on antihypertensive drug therapy, you've got to keep taking those pills for the rest of your life or pay the mortal consequences.

More recently, however, some researchers have been reappraising this theory—especially in light of the financial burden placed on blood pressure sufferers by the ever-increasing cost of the drugs and the potential toxic effects of some of these drugs as they build up in the body over the years.

And in an important study, the antihypertensive-medication-for-life theory took it on the chin. The study, conducted by Northwestern University and Mt. Sinai Hospital in Minneapolis, showed that nearly two-thirds of 90 patients who were eased off their medication—at the same time that they instituted some basic lifestyle changes—still had normal blood pressure after a year-and-a-half. These people had "mild" hypertension with diastolic readings of between 90 and 104 (stage 1 to stage 2 hypertension). An interesting P.S. to the study is that even those whose blood pressure couldn't be held down without returning them to medication were able to maintain normal pressure with dosages lower than before the study.

A study from the Hypertension Detection and Follow-up Program at the University of Mississippi School of Medicine showed pretty much the same results and concluded that mildly hypertensive people (stage 1 to stage 2) whose blood pressure is being controlled by one drug and who are willing to modify their diets are prime candidates for a program involving the elimination of that drug.

Q: So what's the bottom line?

A: Remember, nothing about blood pressure and its treatment is definitive. But the studies seem to indicate that it's possible to be weaned off pressure-lowering medication with impressive results, if you're also willing to lose some weight, stop smoking, lower sodium and alcohol intake and exercise more.

Q: It almost sounds like now we're talking about "stepping down" the care? Is that right?

A: Right. The conclusion follows the stepped care approach that we mentioned in the beginning of this section—first you begin and maintain lifestyle modifications, step up—or shuffle sideways—then (if at all possible) you step down the high-blood-pressure-medication staircase.

Needless to say, it would be unwise to do this on your own initiative, without first discussing the pros and cons with your health-care practitioner.

Q: Very interesting. What else?

A: The big news is that a growing number of medical people (but still, probably and unfortunately, a minority) are joining with mainstream organizations like the American Heart Association and the U.S. government's National Heart, Lung and Blood Institute in the belief that the key to therapy lies not in removing drugs once they've been started, but rather in not prescribing them in the first place—especially for people diagnosed as having mild (stage 1 to stage 2) hypertension.

These doctors and researchers suggest that no study has made a strong case for the use of drugs in what had been called "uncomplicated" mild high blood pressure. What complicates matters are other cardiovascular risk factors muddying up the hypertension waters—things like smoking, diabetes, high cholesterol levels, family history, gender (males are more at risk) and race (African Americans are in greater danger than whites). These factors may add up to a need for some sort of drug therapy. But for most stage 1 to stage 2 hypertension, there's no urgency to rush into pill popping.

Your medical practitioner might not be up on her reading, and might not be following this latest move away from the knee-jerk prescribing. It *isn't* impolite, rude, obnoxious or out of place to bring up these matters. After all, *you* are the one taking—or not taking—the pills.

If your practitioner prescribes any blood pressure medication, find out exactly how and when to take the drug and what side effects, adverse reactions and contraindications are associated with it. Consult drug information books, such as the *PDR Family Guide to Prescription Drugs* or the *Physicians' Desk Reference,* which you should find in your local library. (See Suggested Reading at the back of the book for additional sources.)

Q: What if my blood pressure doesn't improve after trying lifestyle modifications, different medications, combinations of drugs or the strongest dosages?

A: Sadly, some people's blood pressure just can't be controlled, and they die from the disease. Even more sadly, a number of these deaths could be prevented because the failure is not in the drug but in the person taking it—or, rather, not taking it. In many cases, worsened conditions and fatalities are the result of people not taking their medication or not taking it in the proper manner.

If, however, a person is complying with the drug regimen and the blood pressure is still high, it is quite possibly a case of overlooked secondary hypertension, and the physician ought to redouble her efforts to discover the underlying physical cause of the problem.

Q: Can high blood pressure be cured surgically?

A: When kidney troubles are at the root of the problem, surgery to unblock blocked renal arteries or transplants to give the body a healthy kidney often do the job, as do other procedures.

Q: Even though a low blood pressure reading is desirable, when is blood pressure too low? And what are the dangers of **low blood pressure?**

A: The medical term for low blood pressure is **hypotension**, and according to at least one doctor, writing in the *New England Journal of Medicine*, "hypotension is not a disease; it is an ideal blood pressure level." Furthermore, a cardiologist was quoted in the *British Medical Journal* as saying that "the distribution of blood pressure in the population is such that a small percentage of people will have blood pressures well below the mean of the general population." In fact, the Framingham study showed that, as a general rule, the lower the blood pressure, the longer you'll live (although the risk of cardiovascular disease is, oddly enough, somewhat higher for people with diastolic pressure around 70 mm Hg than for those with diastolic pressure around 90 mm Hg).

So long as you feel well with low blood pressure, it's okay. Hypotension does, however, go hand-in-hand with various illnesses and conditions, including diabetes, **Addison's disease** and alcoholism. You can get sudden hypotension (leading to **syncope**—fainting—or even death) after exercise—which might be an indicator of undiscovered heart problems—or after spending time in a sauna. Hypotension may accompany shock.

Orthostatic, or postural, hypotension is a condition—sometimes leading to fainting—that occurs in many people when they sit or stand up suddenly after they've been lying down or sitting for a long time, especially after a stretch in a sick bed. This type of hypotension, as well as the others, may have physical disorders as their root cause. However, they may also be **iatrogenic** in nature; that is, many people suffer hypotension because they'd had hypertension and had begun taking medication—and the medication brought their blood pressure down too low too fast...low enough to cause hypotensive stroke and death.

Q: When is a blood pressure reading considered low blood pressure?

A: Again, it's a smudged line, but a person with low blood pressure is probably getting persistent readings of around 100/70 mm Hg or less.

Q: What can I do about my hypotension?

A: As we said, if you feel all right, you don't have to do anything. If you don't feel all right, get yourself a checkup to see if the hypotension is indicative of a hidden condition. If you're on blood pressure medication, your physician ought to look into reducing the dosage. Ironically, you may have to do the very opposite of what people with high blood pressure should do—you may be urged by your health-care practitioner to add more salt to your diet. If your problem is ortho-static, or postural, in nature, and blood doesn't reach your brain because it's pooling in your legs, you might want to start wearing tight, full-length, elastic support stockings.

Q: Are there any other nonmedical approaches to blood pressure treatment?

A: Beyond the ones we've already talked about—diet, exercise and behavior modification—there are a variety of methods put forth by a variety of nonphysician practitioners and alternative healers. While many of these practitioners can't produce the years of studies and double-blind experimental results that the medical professionals can, they nonetheless provide treatment—often less invasive, less costly and with fewer side effects than traditional medicine's—that has its adherents and success stories.

It's an area of practice unfortunately loaded with charlatans and worse who are out to give unsuspecting sick and desperate people a financial soaking—but it is also an area of therapy that includes some dedicated people, some interesting ideas and some novel approaches. But be careful: Interesting ideas and novel approaches do not necessarily make Jack a well boy. Beware of high prices, unusual and gimmicky machines allegedly designed to undo what's wrong with you, grandiose claims and other things that smack of snake-oil salesmanship. So, caveat emptor—buyer beware—a piece of good old Latin advice, to be applied equally when dealing with medical professionals as well.

Q: With that warning in mind, what are some of the options available in alternative medicine?

A: Nonphysician treatment takes in a lot of territory—from acupuncture (practiced by both

M.D.'s and non-M.D.'s with some good results) to zone therapy, or reflexology, a type of treatment that uses massage of hands and feet to influence the health and function of internal organs and systems.

A number of chiropractors feel that certain blockages of nerves responsible for normal circulation can be eliminated through manipulation techniques.

Practitioners of various massage methods—acupressure and shiatsu chief among them—report that some benefit is derived from their craft, if only that of rubbing away some tension and stress. Homeopathy, which is gaining in popularity and professional favor these days, provides reasonable, limited-invasive treatment through administration of very small doses of homeopathic drugs, salts and elements, in the belief that a tiny amount of the "hair of the dog" that bit you will undo the damage.

Herbalists or herbologists approach the treatment of high blood pressure by prescribing doses of traditionally used flowers, leaves and stems of a large number of plants, often prepared in the form of teas and other beverages.

Hypnotism is coming into its own as a very powerful tool. Through suggestions, much stress-related blood pressure can be eliminated. The same goes for imaging, the creation of pictures or scenarios in your mind to help you actively think the problem away via the mind-body connection. These approaches have slowly moved from the fringe to adjunct positions in the medical bag of therapies.

Doctors of so-called natural healing techniques—naturopaths—may incorporate many of the aforementioned treatments in their practices, along with megavitamin therapy and other nutritional advice. One of this discipline's longtime favorite remedies—eating lots of garlic—has been embraced (at least tentatively) by medical science as a high blood pressure curative and preventive agent.

The gentle, slightly cerebral exercise routines of yoga and tai chi help reduce blood pressure by taking the steam out of stress.

And there are many practitioners—medical and nonmedical alike—who contend that many incidents of high blood pressure are the result of food allergies, and finding and treating the allergy will end the hypertension.

Q: **With so many options, and some possible pitfalls, how do I go about choosing the right alternative method for me?**

A: It's definitely a crowded field and a multifaceted one. Only experience, word-of-mouth recommendations or a good deal of background research can help you to select the method that's best for you . . . if any are. It's a field that lacks consistency—finding two practitioners in the same discipline who will prescribe the same treatment for the very same condition is difficult; they promote their own tried-and-true "sure things"—and it's a field that lacks the consistent reproducibility of results so important to making healing crafts credible. Still, people swear by them and get well by them, and that's as much or more than can be said about conventional medicine.

For people unhappy with the traditional medical approach, these alternatives are available for consideration. Many of them lend themselves to continued self-care too.

Q: So what's the bottom line on all this—by lowering my blood pressure and keeping it low, do I save money in the long run?

A: And in the short run. In addition to doctor visits, the resultant bills, lost work days and medication costs, people with high blood pressure who don't do anything about it pay higher life and health insurance premiums. According to the publication *Medical Economics,* the premium on a five-year term policy for a 35-year-old man may be $847 a year if he's moderately hypertensive, compared with $410 if his blood pressure is normal. People with high blood pressure pay 15 to 25 percent more for health insurance. And it just doesn't make sense, since 95 percent of insurance companies say they'll lower your premium if you drop your high blood pressure to normal for up to two years.

But the real bottom line is your health—and that's something no money can buy.

INFORMATIONAL AND MUTUAL-AID GROUPS

American Heart Association
7272 Greenville Ave.
Dallas, TX 75231
214-373-6300

Coronary Club, Inc.
(Publishes the newletter *Heartline*)
9500 Euclid Ave., EE37
Cleveland, OH 44195
216-444-3690

High Blood Pressure Information Center
120/80 National Institutes of Health
Bethesda, MD 20205

National Hypertension Association
324 E. 30th St.
New York, NY 10016
212-889-3557

National Institute of Hypertension Studies
13217 Livernois
Detroit, MI 48238-3162
313-931-3427

GLOSSARY

Accelerated hypertension: A particularly severe stage of high blood pressure. It is considered a medical emergency (blood pressure readings are quite high, especially the diastolic) that is often fatal in a very short time if left untreated. Related to kidney disease—either as cause or result—accelerated hypertension is a major cause of stroke.

ACE inhibitors: See **angiotensin-converting-enzyme (ACE) inhibitors**.

Addison's disease: A chronic condition in which insufficient amounts of adrenocortical hormone are produced by the adrenal cortex; incurable but controllable through replacement of deficient hormones. Addison's disease symptoms include a general feeling of weakness and fatigue, hypoglycemia, gastrointestinal problems and insufficient cardiac output. Mental and emotional problems also result.

Aerobic exercise: A type of vigorous physical activity designed to improve the body's intake and utilization of oxygen. It is considered excellent exercise for improving cardiovascular health and as a possible preventive of heart attacks and high blood pressure.

Alpha-adrenergic blocking drugs: A class of antihypertensive medications that works through the autonomic nervous system by blocking alpha nerve receptors that normally constrict the blood vessels.

Alpha blockers: See **alpha-adrenergic blocking drugs**.

Ambulatory monitoring: Technique in which a monitor takes multiple blood pressure readings over an extended period of time while a person conducts his or her normal activities.

Angiotensin converting enzyme (ACE) inhibitors: A class of antihypertensive medications that blocks the production of angiotensin, a chemical the body produces to raise blood pressure.

Arterioles: Tiny vessels of arterial circulation that form part of the capillaries. Their muscular walls narrow and widen in response to chemicals made by nerves, so they play an important role in blood vessel resistance and in controlling blood pressure.

Arteriosclerosis: This is a degenerative condition caused by accumulation of minerals and fatty deposits in the arteries, causing a rigidity and inflexibility that affect the flow of blood through the body. In arteriosclerosis, these deposits accumulate in the middle layer of the wall of the artery. Possible causes of arteriosclerosis are high cholesterol levels in the blood, high blood pressure (which, in turn, is worsened by the continued thickening of the deposits and the ever-narrowing path for adequate blood flow), heredity and stress, among others. Commonly known as "hardening of the arteries." See also **atherosclerosis**.

Atherosclerosis: The most prevalent form of arteriosclerosis in which the mineral and fatty deposits accumulate in the inner lining of the walls of the arteries. Atherosclerosis is the major cause of stroke and heart attack in the United States.

Beta-adrenergic blocking drugs: A class of antihypertensive medications that reduces high blood pressure by reducing the force and speed of the heartbeat.

Beta blockers: See **beta-adrenergic blocking drugs**.

Biofeedback: Information provided by various tools and methods that tells a person about any one or several body functions, the goal of which is to teach the person how to control those functions for better health. Biofeedback technology allows a person to hear or see his or her heartbeat or blood pressure or brain waves. Along with expert instruction, that person can then learn to relax, become conscious of those physical states and alter them.

Blood pressure: The force of the blood's journey from the heart to and through the arterial vascular system, and the pressure of the blood expelled from the heart against the walls of the blood vessels it passes through.

Blood pressure cuff: An apparatus involved in taking a blood pressure measurement. See **sphygmomanometer**.

Brachial artery: The artery running down the length of the arm; under ordinary circumstances, it is used to help attain blood pressure measurements through use of the blood pressure cuff.

Calcium channel blockers: A class of antihypertensive medications that works by relaxing the arteries and reducing resistance to the flow of blood.

Cardiac output: A measurement of the volume of blood expelled by a ventricle of the heart. It is usually talked about in terms of volume of blood per minute.

Cardiovascular disease: The many and various diseases affecting the heart and blood vessels. See also **arteriosclerosis, atherosclerosis, congestive heart failure, coronary-artery disease, heart attack, stroke.**

Catecholamines: Chemicals produced by the body that affect the way the body responds to stressful situations. By increasing cardiac output and constricting blood vessels, they work to increase the blood pressure. The best known catecholamines are dopamine, epinephrine and norepinephrine.

Congestive heart failure: A group of conditions involving a weak and failing heart and congestion, usually in the lungs. High blood pressure is a chief cause of congestive heart failure.

Coronary-artery disease: Conditions and diseases involving the arteries that supply blood and oxygen to the heart.

Diastolic: That measurement of blood pressure when the heart is in its resting or relaxation phase, just before the next heartbeat. It is the "lower number" in a blood pressure reading; in a reading of 120/80, for example, the diastolic pressure is indicated by the 80.

Diuretic: A class of drugs that promotes urination, thus speeding the elimination of sodium and water from the body. This is a prescribed method of blood pressure control.

Essential hypertension: A form of hypertension that makes up about 85 to 95 percent of all high blood pressure cases. The cause is unknown—any one of many factors, including heredity and age, may be involved together or separately in affecting the way the body regulates pressure in the arteries. It can be controlled but not cured. Also called primary hypertension.

Heart attack: A popular term for a destructive, often fatal seizure involving the heart. Medical names for this "cardiac event" are *coronary thrombosis* and *myocardial infarction.* Both describe situations wherein a clot (occlusion) of some sort blocks up an artery, thus preventing blood to flow in its normal fashion. This, then, leads to the damage or death of heart muscle.

High blood pressure: See **hypertension.**

High normal blood pressure: A blood pressure level characterized by a systolic reading between 130 and 139 mm Hg and a diastolic reading between 85 and 89 mm Hg.

Hypertension: A disease involving persistent high readings of blood pressure measurement; in general, when readings are taken over a period of time and show blood pressure greater than 140 mm Hg systolic and/or 90 mm Hg diastolic.

Hypertensive heart disease: A disorder that occurs in people with high blood pressure when the heart, forced to work harder to pump blood through narrowed blood vessels, becomes enlarged. The pumping action of the heart is affected, and circulatory failure follows.

Hypotension: Low blood pressure. A person is usually considered hypotensive if he or she has continual blood pressure readings in which the systolic reading is less than 100 mm Hg and/or the diastolic reading is less than 70 mm Hg.

Iatrogenic: Description of diseases or conditions that occur because of the actions of a physician or another health-care professional. Doctor-caused illnesses are the result of iatrogenesis.

Isometric exercise: A form of physical activity and body-building that involves the application of bodily force against stable resistance.

Labile hypertension: High blood pressure that fluctuates and is not persistent. If untreated, labile hypertension can become persistent and health endangering. See also **sustained hypertension**.

Left ventricle: A chamber of the heart on the lower left side. It pumps oxygenated blood into the circulatory system and body tissues.

Low blood pressure: See **hypotension**.

Malignant hypertension: See **accelerated hypertension**.

Mild hypertension: A blood pressure level characterized by a diastolic reading between 90 and 104 mm Hg, according to an older medical classification system. See **stage 1** and **stage 2 hypertension**.

Moderate hypertension: A blood pressure level characterized by a diastolic reading between 105 and 114 mm Hg, according to an older medical classification system. See **stage 2** and **stage 3 hypertension**.

Normal blood pressure: A blood pressure level with a systolic reading between 120 and 129 mm Hg and a diastolic reading between 80 and 84.

Normotensive: A term to describe a person whose blood pressure falls into normal, acceptable limits.

Optimal blood pressure: A systolic blood pressure reading less than 120 mm Hg and a diastolic reading less than 80 mm Hg.

Peripheral adrenergic antagonists: This drug class dilates blood vessels by inhibiting the release of adrenaline, resulting in lowered blood pressure.

Peripheral vasodilators: A type of antihypertensive drug that works by opening the blood vessels to decrease resistance to blood flow.

Primary hypertension: See **essential hypertension**.

Prostacyclin: A chemical in the body that acts as a vaso-dilator; that is, a blood vessel opener.

Pulse pressure: A figure that indicates the difference between the systolic pressure and the diastolic pressure.

Renal artery stenosis: A narrowing or obstruction of the kidney's artery.

Retina: A membrane at the back of the eye that receives the images passed into the eye through the lens and sends them, via the optic nerve, to the brain. It is the only place in the human body where the arteries and arterioles can be looked at directly to see if any damage indicative of hypertension exists.

Secondary hypertension: High blood pressure caused by some underlying disease or ailment. By eliminating the physical cause of secondary hypertension—for example, a kidney problem—it is often possible to bring the elevated blood pressure back to normal. In this way, it is unlike primary (essential) hypertension, which has no discernible cause.

Severe hypertension: A blood pressure level characterized by a diastolic reading above 115 mm Hg, according to an older medical classification system. See **stage 3** and **stage 4 hypertension**.

Sleep apnea: An occasional, temporary stoppage of breathing while asleep, as a result of a failure of the autonomic nervous system to regulate the breathing. It leads to several conditions, among them high blood pressure.

Sphygmomanometer: The device most commonly used to measure systolic and diastolic blood pressures. It allows notation and comparison of blood pressure levels by giving those values on a scale measured in millimeters (mm) of mercury (Hg).

Stage 1 hypertension: A blood pressure level characterized by a systolic reading between 140 and 159 mm Hg and a diastolic reading between 90 and 99 mm Hg.

Stage 2 hypertension: A blood pressure level characterized by a systolic reading between 160 and 179 mm Hg and a diastolic reading between 100 and 109 mm Hg.

Stage 3 hypertension: A blood pressure level characterized by a systolic reading between 180 and 209 mm Hg and a diastolic reading between 110 and 119 mm Hg.

Stage 4 hypertension: A blood pressure level characterized by a systolic reading greater than 210 mm Hg or a diastolic reading greater than 120 mm Hg.

Stepped care: A method of antihypertensive therapy that begins with lifestyle modifications and moves into a low dose of a family of drugs, building up dosage gradually in that and other drugs until control of pressure is achieved.

Stroke: A cerebrovascular accident wherein a ruptured or blocked blood vessel prevents blood from reaching important portions of the brain, leading to brain damage and subsequent debilitating conditions, including paralysis and often death.

Sustained hypertension: A description of high blood pressure that stays at the same high levels all the time and does not fluctuate to any important degree. See also **labile hypertension.**

Syncope: Fainting, as a result of insufficient blood flow to the brain.

Systolic: That measurement of blood pressure when the left ventricle contracts and the blood's force against the vessel walls is at its greatest strength. It is the higher number in a blood pressure reading; that is, in a reading of 120/80, for example, the systolic pressure is indicated by the 120.

Thiazide: A type of diuretic that works to reduce sodium, chloride and water levels in the body through increased urination.

Tinnitus: A ringing, buzzing, roaring or some other sort of noise in the ears that is long-term, distracting, dismaying and often debilitating.

Vascular system: The body's network of blood vessels.

Vasopressin: A hormone stored in the pituitary gland which, when released, causes the capillaries and arterioles to contract, resulting in an elevation of blood pressure.

Vertigo: A sensation that makes a person feel as though either he or the world is spinning dizzily. It is often caused by high blood pressure or diseases of the inner ear, among other causes.

White-coat hypertension: The tendency for blood pressure to increase in the presence of a physician.

SUGGESTED READING

Barrow, Mark V. *Heart Talk: Understanding Cardiovascular Diseases.* Gainesville, Fla.: Cor-Ed Publishing Co., 1992.

Braunwald, Eugene. *Heart Disease: A Textbook of Cardiovascular Medicine.* 3rd ed. Philadelphia: W.B. Saunders Company, 1988.

Budnick, Herbert N. *Heart to Heart: A Guide to the Psychological Aspects of Heart Disease.* Ann Arbor, Mich.: Health Administrative Press, 1994.

Cooper, Kenneth. *Controlling Cholesterol: Preventive Medicine Program.* New York: Bantam, 1989.

Diethrich, Edward B., and Carol Cohan. *Women & Heart Disease: What You Can Do to Stop the Number-One Killer of American Women.* New York: Ballantine, 1994.

Douglas, Pamela S., ed. *Cardiovascular Health & Disease in Women.* Philadelphia: W.B. Saunders Company, 1993.

Hellerstein, Herman, and Paul Perry. *Healing Your Heart: A Proven Program for Lowering Cholesterol and Preventing or Healing Heart Disease.* New York: Simon & Schuster, 1990.

Horovitz, Emmanuel. *Cholesterol Control Made Easy: How to Lower Your Cholesterol for a Healthier Heart.* Encino, Calif.: Health Trend, 1990.

Jones, Paul, M.D., and Angela Mitchell. *The Black Health Library Guide to Heart Disease and Hypertension.* New York: Henry Holt & Co., 1993.

Karpman, Harold L. *Preventing Silent Heart Disease: Detecting and Preventing America's Number 1 Killer.* New York: Crown, 1989.

Khan, M. Gabriel. *Heart Attacks, Hypertension and Heart Drugs.* Emmaus, Pa.: Rodale, 1986.

Lowen, Alexander. *Love, Sex & Your Heart.* New York: Viking Penguin, 1994.

Mayo Clinic Staff. *Mayo Clinic Heart Book.* New York: William Morrow & Co., 1993.

Medical Economics Data. *The PDR Family Guide to Prescription Drugs.* Montvale, N.J.: Medical Economics Data, 1995.

Medical Economics Data. *Physicians' Desk Reference.* Montvale, N.J.: Medical Economics Data, 1996.

Ornish, Dean, M.D. *Dr. Dean Ornish's Program for Reversing Heart Disease.* New York: Random House, 1990.

Pashkow, Frederick, and Charlotte Libove. *The Woman's Heart Book: The Complete Guide to Keeping Your Heart Healthy and What to Do If Things Go Wrong.* New York: Dutton, 1993.

Pierce, James B., Ph.D. *Heart Health Magnesium.* Garden City Park, N.Y.: Avery Publishing Group, 1994.

Prevention Magazine Staff, eds. *Lower Your Blood Pressure: Controlling Your Blood Pressure Without Drugs.* Stamford, Conn.: Longmeadow Press, 1991.

Villarosa, Linda, ed. *Body & Soul: The Black Women's Guide to Physical Health and Emotional Well-Being.* New York: HarperCollins, 1994.

Wikman-Coffelt, Joan. *Your Heart: A Battery for Life.* Pittsburgh: Dorrance Publishing Co., 1994.

Zaret, Barry L., M.D., Marvin Moses, M.D., and Lawrence S. Cohen, M.D. *Yale University School of Medicine Heart Book.* New York: Hearst Books, 1992.

INDEX

Locators followed by a t indicate tables.

life/health insurance and, 82
malignant, 26, 88
mild, 20, 88
moderate, 20, 88
obesity and, 42-43
primary. *See* Essential
hypertension
reduction, 25-26, 32
salt and, 35, 48-54
seasons and, 31
secondary, 24, 87
severe, 20, 89
smoking and, 30, 39-40
stage 1, 21, 89
stage 2, 21, 89
stage 3, 21, 89
stage 4, 21, 90
stress and, 33-34, 35, 80, 81
sustained, 15, 90
symptoms, 22-23
treatment
alternative medicine, 79-81
drug companies and, 65-66
drug therapy. *See* specific
medications
lifestyle modification, 63
weather and, 31
white-coat, 14, 27-28, 90
Hypertensive heart disease, 25, 87
Hypnotism, 80
Hypotension, 77-78, 87

I

Iatrogenic, 78, 88
Inderal. *See* Beta-adrenergic
blocking drugs
Informational and mutual-aid
groups, 83
Insurance, hypertension and, 82
Inversion therapy, 38
Isometric exercise, 37, 88
Isradipine. *See* Calcium channel
blockers

K

Kidney disease, 21, 24, 76
Kidney surgery, 76

L

Labile hypertension, 15, 88
Lasix. *See* Furosemide
Left ventricle, 9, 88
Lisinopril. *See* Angiotensin-
converting enzyme (ACE)
inhibitors
Lopressor. *See* Beta-adrenergic
blocking drugs
Low blood pressure, 77. *See also*
Hypotension

M

Magnesium, 54, 56-57, 56t, 57t
Malignant hypertension, 26, 88
Meditation, 35
Metoprolol. *See* Beta-adrenergic
blocking drugs
Mild hypertension, 20, 88
Minipress. *See* Alpha-adrenergic
blocking drugs
Moderate hypertension, 20, 88
MSG, sodium content, 52-53

N

Nadolol. *See* Beta-adrenergic
blocking drugs
Natriuretic hormone, 21
Naturopathy, 80-81
Nervousness, 33-34
Nicotine. *See* Smoking
Nifedipine. *See* Calcium channel
blockers
Normal blood pressure, 11, 20,
27t, 88
Normotensive, 49, 88
Nosebleeds, 23

O

Obesity, 42-43
Olive oil, 45
Omega-3 fatty acids, 46
Optimal blood pressure, 20, 27t, 88
Oral contraceptives, 29-30, 40

P

Peripheral adrenergic antagonists,
71, 88